How to Live a Healthier and Younger

Looking Life

By

Okongor Ayuk Ndifon

Usage:

You may use this ebook without giving it out and without selling it.

DISCLAIMER AND/OR LEGAL NOTICES:

The information presented herein represents author's view as of the date of publication.

Due to the fact that the rate with which conditions change, with the use of the internet, the author reserves the right to alter and update his opinion based on the new conditions.

It is hoped that the knowledge gained from this ebook would go along way to helping you adapt to the changing condition of the internet.

The ebook is for information purposes only. While every attempt has been made to verify the information provided in this ebook, the author assume any

CONTENT

Introduction

How to live a healthier and younger looking life is actually a combination of two volumes into one volume or book.

The book arose from the fact that many people know little about their health, youthfulness, and aging process.

Many people think that life is what you see and cannot do anything to improve on it, but rather to suffer whatever state you find yourself in.

They never mind seeking, caring, and curing minor or major diseases that come their way, and even fail to seize on the beauty of nature to live and maintain a healthier, and younger looking life.

It cannot be denied that fact that other people may not fall sick, but age is taking a toll on them. This is seen by the presence of wrinkles, grey hair, high fatigue, obesity, and inactivity.

Even though doctors, dermatologists, health, and beauty personnel abound, many are unable to reach out to them due to one reason or the other.

It therefore becomes imperative for this book, How to live a healthier and Younger Looking life.

With this book, you can easily study what might be the cause, prevention, and cure measures for any of the treated ailments that may plague your body, even before or after seeing your doctor.

Doing so, will help you prevent and combat many diseases and conditions that may come your way.

Using the information in this book and applying what you learn, can help you live a healthier, happier, and younger looking life.

CHAPTER 1

SOME RECURRING DISEASES

S ome diseases keep recurring on a regular basis among the various complaints and diagnoses in medicine. But with a good understanding and better approaches of prevention and control, they can be subdued.

i. Heart Diseases, Prevention, and Management

U nderstanding the different types of heart diseases and knowing if you have risk factors can help you to prevent being diagnosed with it.

Heart disease is the number one killer in developed nations and a major cause of disability. It often exists for a long time without any symptoms. Such heart diseases include:

1. Heart valve diseases or valvular heart disease

The heart has four valves that let blood flow into or out of the heart for normal functioning of the heart, and close to hinder blood flowing back.

Problem arises when they do not function properly, leading to leakage of blood, and resulting in what is called regurgitation.

Mitral valve prolapsed, is a problem or disease of the heart valve, where the mitral valve becomes flaps that are unable to close fully.

Another condition called stenosis occurs when the valves do not open adequately, thereby hindering blood flow.

Heart valve diseases may be present at birth and some need no treatment, while some require repair through surgery.

2. High Blood Pressure

High blood pressure, also called hypertension, is the constant elevation of the pressure of blood pushing against the walls of the arteries and other blood vessels.

Blood pressure is the force of imported blood on the walls of the arteries. This force is brought about by the heart as a result of its pumping of blood to all parts of the body.

High blood pressure usually manifest in middle age. Periodic checks, medical advice, prescribed medication from your doctor can bring about prevention and cure.

3. Cardiac Arrhythmia

Cardiac arrhythmia is a heart condition in which the heart goes off-beat. Here the heart beat rate may become lower or higher than normal. It can result to other heart problem.

4. Coronary Artery Disease

The disease is also called coronary arteriosclerosis or coronary atherosclerosis. This disease occur when the arteries that give blood to the heart become blocked or hardened and smaller or narrow, due to bad cholesterol and other harmful materials buildup on the inner walls.

The heart at this time cannot receive the needed blood. Signs and symptoms include pain in the chest. This can lead to other heart diseases like heart attack. See your doctor for help.

5. Heart Attack

Also known as cardiac failure is a condition whereby the heart is unable to pump blood round the body in a way in which it uses to do. This may result to blood backup in ankles, feet, etc. The weakness of the heart results in this.

Signs and symptoms observed are tiredness, and shortness of breath. Cure includes heart transplant, medication, and medical help.

6. Rheumatic Heart disease and other Infections heart Disease

These diseases are linked with some streptococcal infections. Typhoid, syphilis, diphtheria, tuberculosis, and other fevers can work against the heart and cause harm and disease.

Treatment of these fevers can bring prevention and treatment.

ii. High Blood Pressure

Signs and Preventive Measures for High Blood Pressure

High blood pressure or hypertension is a consistent rise of the pressure of blood, pulsing against the walls of the arteries and other blood vessels.

When in regular blood examination, the blood pressure measurements gives a significant rise above the normal range. When you see signs of high blood pressure, there is the need to seek for preventive measures.

Many factors are responsible for causing high blood pressure. These may be hereditary, endocrine or emotional factors.

Other factors also may play a part in causing high blood pressure. Signs of high blood pressure must be known to enable you detect the underlying cause, so as to apply preventive measures for high blood pressure profitably.

High blood pressure can cause many problems, like kidney disease, heart attack, and stroke. People who are too fat are victims. To be too fat is not healthy.

Too much fat aids in causing high blood pressure, diabetes, gallstones, arthritis, and the above mentioned diseases.

Signs of high blood pressure which would necessitate preventive measures, includes, weakness and dizziness, frequent headaches, pounding of the heart and shortness of breath whenever you engage in a minor exercise or activity.

At the onset of high blood pressure, there appear to be no signs. Signs of high blood pressure are actually when the situation becomes dangerous.

Where signs of high blood pressure abound, there is the need for preventive measures to be taken, to avert the dangerous condition.

Preventive measures for high blood pressure include:

1. Eat balanced diets

Avoid eating fatty, greasy, or oily foods. You must put away sugar or sweet foods. You must also avoid eating too much of carbohydrates, like bread, potatoes, rice, yam, and corn. Use vegetable oil instead of pig fat, and lean meat instead of red meat. You should eat more of fruits and vegetables.

2. Lose your weight, if overweight

If you see that you are overweight, seek to lose your weight immediate to avoid endangering yourself. Your diet should be reduced or halved, to enable you lose weight.

3. Avoid Smoking of cigarette and Drinking of Alcohol

These are harmful habits to your health. Smoking of cigarette and drinking of alcohol are habits that distort the normal functioning of your body, thereby causing diseases and other health problems.

4. Seek Medical Help

When you notice the above signs of high blood pressure, or have an extremely high blood pressure, seek medical help immediately. See your doctor, and take prescribed drugs regularly.

It is possible to lower your high blood pressure, when you have noticed the above signs of high blood pressure, follow the above preventive measures for high blood pressure, and the relief would come.

For some persons, what they need is to lose weight, and their high blood pressure, becomes lowered.

Ways to Reduce Your Risks of High Blood Pressure

This information about high blood pressure or hypertension gives definite ways to reduce your risks of the disease.

Blood pressure refers to the pressure under which blood flows through the arteries. Its level depends on three major factors, the first being, amount of blood in the system.

If the volume of blood circulating in this closed system is reduced, the pressure will drop. In the same vein, if the volume of blood circulating increases, the pressure will rise.

The volume of blood in your circulation will decrease when you suffer a hemorrhage - a loss of blood from injury, an operation, or internal bleeding through peptic ulcer.

If the pressure drops too low, a shock occurs - that is a state of circulatory collapse.

High blood pressure is a risk factor for heart disease, stroke (where blood arteries clog or rupture), blindness - where arteries become blocked, heart attacks, cardiac failure, and aneurysms of the aorta.

The second factor that determines the hearts pumping action is when the heart is weakened during a heart attack or by some other cardiac disease. The third factor affecting your blood pressure level is the tone of the arteries walls.

One factor can increase your risk, especially if combined with other risk factors like being overweight, being sedentary, over consumption of salt, eating to little of potassium, and engaging in high stress levels.

The following ways will help reduce your increased risks of high blood pressure.

1. If you are obese, shed some weight.

Overweight or obese persons are at increased risk of having high blood pressure. It has been estimated that in cases of high blood pressure, being overweight is one major cause.

If overweight is a cause of hypertension, then losing weight is known to lower blood pressure.

2.   Reduce your consumption of salt

It is known that reducing your salt intake or consumption to half is enough to lower blood pressure. Eat no salt or low salt diets, to help you lower blood pressure.

3.   Quit alcohol consumption

People who drink alcohol and alcoholic beverages are known to be more likely to develop high blood pressure than those who do not drink. What alcohol does is to dilate your system and cause high blood pressure. So, quit drinking alcohol.

4.   Eat Bananas for potassium need

Banana is packed with potassium. Potassium as a mineral has been recommended by experts to help increase the level of potassium in those with low potassium levels. Other potassium rich foods recommended for those with hypertension and low potassium intake include tomatoes, potatoes with skins, apricots, prunes, and broccoli.

5.   Avoid Stress, Get Exercise and Relaxation

Do morning or midday workouts. Also, do brisk walking, stationary cycling, or jogging. Exercise should be done for at least 30 minutes daily to help reduce your risks of high blood pressure.

Exercising can help you manage stress. Learn also to relax. Relaxation will help lower pressure in persons suffering

hypertension.

iii. Acute Pericarditis(Heart Problem)

Combating Acute Pericarditis (Heart Problem)

C ombating acute pericarditis and conquering it is a must to be free from this dreaded heart attack. Pericardium is a membrane or sac which holds or covers the heart. Think of it as an apple enclosed in a polythene sac. Pericarditis is a disease or inflammation of the pericardium. The root cause or causes of the inflammation may be due to infection or otherwise.

Signs and Symptoms

In all heart diseases, as well as pericarditis, observable signs and symptoms include:

i.   Breathlessness or shortness of breath after a slight exertion

ii.   Chest pain or tightness

ii.   Swollen legs, ankles or abdomen

iii.   Tiredness without a known origin

iv.   Double vision

v.   Severe and persistent headache

vi.   Dizziness

vii.   Indigestion

viii.   Loss of appetite

ix.   Low or excessive heart beat

x.   Fever, if infected

xi.   Coma, if critical

Pericarditis can result to obstruction in heart pumping, and hindrance to normal muscular heart pump. In this way fluid may collect, leading to heart failure.

Diagnoses require adequate and complete clinical and radiological tests, like scanning, blood analysis, x-ray, ECG, CAT, advanced imaging techniques, etc.

Proper treatment involves knowledge of the patient's history or medical record, both past and present, to find out the true cause of the problem, and to be able to proffer the best treatment possible.

Pericarditis and other heart diseases are serious conditions that may put the life of victims in danger. The condition is best handled by cardiologists in a specialist hospital, with best medical facilities and medical experts.

The heart may be operated. Heart operations have been known to occur in cases of joint heart, hole in the heart, Siamese twins, and in the insertion of pacemaker in the heart for better heart pumping. Cardiac heart transplant may be administered, as a form of treatment to bring relief.

Cardiologist or medical experts can help any victim of acute pericarditis by maintaining circulation with cardiac support machines, undertaking frequent ECG and diagnosis, control and cure of infections.

Other expert help include: administering quality drugs, cross matching blood perfectly, keeping the kidneys in good condition, being careful with drips, observe adequate monitoring, and watchfulness. Early treatment of infections that may result to acute pericarditis, can offer help.

In addition, moderate diet, personal hygiene, and exercise, must be considered before this time.

Harmful habits like alcohol intake, cigarette and smoking, should be avoided. Stress level must be managed favorably too, with adequate rest, and freedom from anxiousness.

Good Food for a Healthy Heart

Good food for a healthy heart depends on what you eat. Agents responsible for blood vessel damage, cause heart disease.

Oxygen in a place where it is not supposed to be found can cause a tendency for it to react with fatty substances and turn them into harmful compounds.

These oxidized fats can cause clogging of arteries. Oxidized fats get into the body through two means, in diets or when oxygen reacts with fats in your body.

It is important to cut down on dietary fats, to be able to limit your intake of oxidized fats, and reduce the circulation of fats in your blood after a meal.

You must eat fewer fried foods, to be able to effectively lower your blood cholesterol.

Although, oxidized fats cannot be totally avoided, your body has the ability to prevent fat from being oxidized, and neutralizes fat that would have reacted with oxygen.

To be able to get your body to have this defense mechanism, your body needs a daily supply of antioxidants from your diets.

The following antioxidant nutrients with their food sources will help you get the best in having a healthy heart.

1. Vitamin A: Sources of vitamin A are beta-carotene, egg yolk, and liver.

2. Vitamin C: Sources include peppers, broccoli, citrus, melons, berries, and tropical fruits.

3. Vitamin E: Sources include nuts, wheat germ, seeds and their oils.

4. Beta-carotene: sources include sweet potatoes, apricots, paw-paw, and dark yellow and green vegetables.

5. Selenium: sources include: Red meat, whole grains, nuts, and sea foods.

6. Zinc: Sources include whole grains, oysters, liver, and sea foods.

You must avoid high fat ingredients, including butter, oil, cream, and sour cream.

Also, avoid high fat foods like cheese, sausage, and avocado, and high fat cooking methods like broiling with butter, frying, and sauntering.

Endeavor to watch your cholesterol level, by consuming less saturated fat, from foods like full fat yogurt, cheese, whole milk, and sour cream; and less Trans fat present in fried and processed foods. It is recommended to eat more of fish.

Avoid high oil and sodium diets, and make sure you cut down on these by eating steamed rice instead of fried.

Also, avoid egg rolls, fried dumplings, and higher fat diets like pork. In addition avoid deep fried chicken and fish.

This is so because there are many problems involved with fried food, as they are not good food for a healthy heart. If you desire a healthy heart, eat good foods as outlined above.

Heart diseases can be prevented or managed or treated by knowing underlying causes, avoiding harmful habits like smoking, dealing with bad cholesterol, having adequate exercise daily, having a stress free life, and seeing your doctor.

iv. High Cholesterol

Simple Steps to Lower High cholesterol

High cholesterol is dangerous to your health, but there are simple steps to lower the condition. We have good cholesterol and bad cholesterol that can occur in a body.

The good one is good for your body, while the bad cholesterol or high cholesterol is bad for your health.

Good cholesterol enables the building of essential hormones and healthy cells. Clogging of fats takes place in your body in the presence of high cholesterol in your blood system.

This causes blockage of your arteries, making it hard for your heart to get oxygenated blood, which you need for your normal body function. You may have heart attack as a result of this problem. Many people suffer stroke as a result of this problem too.

How can you lower and treat your high cholesterol level? Follow the simple steps below:

1. Understand factors that Causes High Cholesterol

Risk factors are associated with this problem. There are two types of risk factors. These are uncontrollable and controllable risk factors.

A. Controllable factors include:

i. Consumption of saturated fats and cholesterol foods.

This raises the total cholesterol level.

ii. Becoming or Being Overweight

B. Uncontrollable factors include:

i. Age.

Men who are 45 years or above, and women who are 35 years and above, have increased risk of high cholesterol

ii. Gender

This applies to women only. This occurs after menopause.

iii. Your family History

If mother, father, sister, and brother, have had cases of hearth attack at certain ages, it becomes possible that it runs in the blood line

2. Undergo a Test

Your blood can be diagnosed in the medical laboratory, to determined whether you have high cholesterol

3. Lower and Treat your High Cholesterol

It is possible to lower and treat high cholesterol. We have two ways of lowering high cholesterol.

a. Change or Modify Your Diet

Eat balanced diets to be able to lower your high cholesterol. The diets are called medical nutrition therapy.

Consult a doctor for this special diet. The diet includes advice on the total fat and saturated fat to eat daily.

b. Avoid or Quit Smoking

Smoking causes bad cholesterol to form in your arteries. Smoking also increases the risk of heart disease

c. You must lose weight

Being overweight is a risk factor. Losing weight can help to lower your high cholesterol.

d. Engage in Regular Exercise

Experts' advice that you exercise for a minimum of 30 - 45 minutes for about five to six days of a week

It is important that you exercise and lose weight, because these would increase your good cholesterol and lower you bad cholesterol.

e. Medication

If you can not lower your high cholesterol to acceptable or desirable levels through change of life style, your doctor may prescribe medication, to go hand in hand with your new diet and exercise program.

V. Overcoming Osteoarthritis and Arthritis

Maintaining a Healthy Cartilage to Avoid Osteoarthritis

It is necessary to maintain a healthy cartilage in order to avoid osteoarthritis.

Osteoarthritis is a cartilage degenerative disease. So, without giving attention to the cartilage, it begins to wear and tear.

There is the need to how to regenerate a degenerative cartilage and the type of nutrition required to have a healthy cartilage.

The three types of joints in the body are covered with a smooth and shiny attachment between the bones, called cartilage.

The cartilage help in the movement of joints, gives protection to the bones, protects the bones from rubbing against one another in order to prevent damage to the joints during movement.

The cartilage is semi-transparent, with no blood vessels and depends on exchange of fluid for its nourishment. The cartilages consist of 80% water.

A healthy cartilage can enable one to take part in sports and other activities without pains. But pains come any time you engage in activities when the cartilage becomes thin and worn out.

Cells of the cartilage may start to die due to toxicity, poor nutrition or systemic disease process. If this process continues the cartilage begins to break and crack. This results to joint degeneration or cartilage degeneration.

Due to wear and tear of the cartilage, enzymes begin will begin to leak into the cartilage, thereby destroying more of the collagen.

This brings about increased joint pain, due to the repetition of joint destruction. This results to the cartilage becoming very thin and worn out in so much that it wears through and exposes the bones.

This can lead to difficulty in repairing the cartilage and causes the body to develop a false cartilage called fibro-cartilage. This type of cartilage has a short lifespan, because it wears out shortly after being developed or formed.

The bones become inflamed, with leakage of fluid into the bones causing more harm to the bones.

You must be able to arrest the situation early enough urgent lifestyle changes, nutritional management, and herbal remedy. This can be done through the following ways:

1.   Take Adequate Quantity of Water Daily

Since the cartilage is made up of 80% of water, it is necessary to give attention to drinking of water, in order to prevent osteoarthritis.

It is recommended that women should drink up to two and half liters of water daily, and men should drink three liters of water daily. It is important to have enough water intakes in order to have enough synovial fluid.

Adequate water intake will bring about a healthy joint and cartilage.

2. Avoiding the Consumption of Certain Foods that Causes inflammation

When you avoid these harmful foods, start eating foods that will energize and renew your cartilage.

Foods with fatty acids found in saturated fats and animal products should be avoided, because they cause inflammation. These include red meat, pork, poultry, egg yolk, and all dairy products other than non-fat dairy products.

Foods rich in omega-6 fatty acid or supplements should be avoided, since inflammation is the main characteristics of rheumatoid arthritis. Make sure that on a daily basis fatty foods intake be reduced or avoided, in order to control inflammation.

Oils rich in omega-6 fatty acids should be avoided. They include corn and sunflower oils, margarine, palm oil, and fried foods. In place of these foods, consume extra virgin olive oil and other foods that are high in mono-saturated fats, which include almonds, and avocados.

Foods rich in omega-3 fatty acids should bee consumed. They are found basically in fatty fish and marine plants.

Fatty fish include salmon, herring, mackerel, tuna, and sardines. Eat foods rich in vitamin B, which includes beans, wheat germs, tuna, alfalfa, salmon, soy beans, peanuts, walnuts, whole wheat, brown rice, and brewer's yeast, etc.

3.   Appropriate Medication

You must consult your doctor for prescription of drugs to take.

Make sure that you involve timely management through lifestyle changes and appropriate medication, to enable a fast and speedy recovery within a short time.

Ways to Prevent and Treat Arthritis

Arthritis is a disease condition which brings about inflammation of the joints and accompanying pains, stiffness, redness, and swelling. The various ways to prevent and treat arthritis are as follows:

1.   Avoid Caffeine Intake

Consumption of coffee on a regular basis can bring about a change in your normal body function. Caffeine is a stimulant. So, if you an arthritis patient, it is better to stay clear from caffeine intake.

2.   Avoid Tobacco Intake

It is known fact that smoking is dangerous to your health. For you to be healed of arthritis, you need to avoid or quit smoking.

3. Reduce salt Intake

Excessive consumption of salt results in many abnormalities including hypertension and arthritis. This is so because excess salt hinders the normal flow of blood to various parts of the body, including the joints.

4. Avoid Sugar and Sugary Foods

White sugar is dangerous to your health. You also need to be careful concerning foods that are packed with sugar. Sugar is capable of causing inflammation in the body and joints, resulting in arthritis.

5. Reduce or Avoid Fat Consumption

Bad fat consumption is dangerous to your health. You must reduce or avoid the use of fatty foods in your diets. Do not consume fatty milk, other dairy products, and red meat.

6. Avoid Eating Oranges and other Citrus Fruits

Oranges and citrus fruits contain uric acid. So, avoid their consumption to avoid uric acid deposit.

7. Eat Fiber, Fruits and Vegetables

Consume some fiber foods, flax seeds, oat bran, beans, and dark green vegetables daily.

Also, eat pineapple frequently. An enzyme found in pineapple helps to reduce inflammation. Avoid eating refrigerated and canned pineapple, but eat fresh pineapple.

8. Consume foods with Histidine Amino Acid

Eat foods containing the amino acid Histidine, including rice, wheat, and rye. Histidine is effective in removing excess metals from the body.

Many people with arthritis have high levels of copper and iron in their bodies.

9. Relief stiffness with a hot shower as against cold shower.

Stiffness due to arthritis can be relieved by having a hot shower instead a cold one.

10.   Make Use of pain relievers

Put salt into kerosene and dab on the affected parts to relief pain. Do not rub on the skin.

Also, relief pain by placing cabbage folds with bandage overnight. Pain can also be relieved by rubbing raw lemon and hot castor oil.

11.   Avoid allergies, take fresh air, and sunlight

12.   Observe regular and moderate exercise

Exercise is important for reducing pains and keeping the body fit and healthy. Regular exercise removes stress on the affected joints. Do jogging, cycling, and swimming exercises regularly. Lose excess weight if you are obese.

As an arthritis patient, take heed to the above ways of preventing and treating arthritis and all shall be well.

Vi. Kidney Troubles Prevention

Preventive Measures against kidney Diseases

Preventing kidney diseases is a must, to be able to stay free from many of the kidney disorders that plague humans, and even leading to general poor health.

Functions of the Kidney

The kidney is a pear-shaped organ that functions mainly for the maintenance of blood volume, excretion of waste materials, maintenance of a stable internal environment of the body, and assistance in red blood cells production. The actual production of red blood cells takes place in the bone marrow, but the kidney produces a chemical called erythropoietin, which enables the bone marrow to produce the red blood cells.

Some organisms and foreign particles get into the body and may cause harm to the body. These foreign invaders into the body are unwanted.

The kidney assists liver in the detoxification of invaded agents and organisms in the body before eliminating them. The body produces chemicals to immobilize these foreign invaders, and the kidney works a way for their elimination out of the body.

The activities of the kidney can cause it to malfunction and become disease infected, which then necessitates preventing kidney diseases.

Causes of kidney Diseases

Foreign invaders and organisms into the body include bacteria, viruses, protozoa fungi infection in any part of the body.

Known infections against the body, these invaders cause are skin infection, bone infections, heart infections, cold, catarrh, sore throat, diarrhea, hepatitis, malaria, and HIV.

Some other causes of kidney diseases include Use of medicated soaps and creams with mercury content, pollution and environmental pollutants from waste from industries, use of lightening creams and soap.

Other causes are tinned food contaminants, drug and herbal abuse, use of fake and adulterated drugs, abnormal body responses to drugs, and toxins from plants.

Body breakdown may be caused by specific diseases like diabetes mellitus, hypertension, urinary tract infection, prostrate enlargement, and some complications of pregnancy, cancer, hereditary and genital abnormalities of the body. The list also includes sickle cell diseases, anemia, severe deprivation of water and excessive sweating or dehydration. You then that the need for preventing kidney diseases cannot be over-emphasized.

Signs and symptoms of kidney Diseases

Signs and symptoms of kidney diseases include difficulties in urinating. Victims may pass out much water or too little water, in a painful or too frequent manner.

Diagnosis or urinalysis may reveal blood, casts, pus, albumin, and other abnormal things in the urine.

Kidney diseases may show up with non-specific symptoms like body aches, headache, and tiredness. These usually come up during common complaints to a doctor.

Another sign of kidney diseases is swelling and puffiness of body tissues, due to accumulation of fluids in them (a condition called edema), backache, and severe pains in the kidneys.

Preventing kidney diseases involves taking care of what you eat and drink, and stopping the use of mercury containing soaps and lightening creams, drug abuse, blood pressure, etc.

vii. Conquering Diabetes

Detection and Management Approaches to Conquer Diabetes

Detection and management approaches to conquer diabetes become necessary when it is known that some victims of diabetes are unable to know that they are diabetic. In addition to the inability to detect their diabetes status, is the need to conquer the disease.

Diabetes mellitus is a disease which occur in an individual due to the inability of his or her body to make use of sugar, due to insulin deficiency.

Insulin is a hormone produced by the pancreas and is essential for the breakdown of carbohydrates or sugar. For energy to be produced, insulin is responsible for speeding the uptake of sugar into the cells.

When insulin is lacking in an individual's blood, diabetes mellitus occurs, in which case the blood sugar level is very high or in excess.

The excess sugar is removed through the kidney and passed out in urine. As such, the presence of sugar in the blood or urine is an indication that one has diabetes mellitus.

Diabetes can result in very serious complication, but with early detection and management approaches, the ailment can be conquered and controlled. If diabetes mellitus is conquered and controlled, victims can live normal lives.

The root cause of diabetes is yet unknown, but there are predisposing factors that may play a role in developing diabetes.

The main factors are hereditary, while others include excessive weight gain or obesity, stress, side effects of certain drugs, and lack of exercise.

Detection of the disease condition takes place through common signs and symptoms. As such, the common signs and symptom of diabetes mellitus include, Frequent urination, Excessive thirst for water or fluids.

Other common signs and symptoms of diabetes are Drinking of large quantities of water and emptying same within a short time, Sexual weakness, Recurrent abortions, Still births, Delivery of bigger than expected babies, Frequent occurrence of boils, pains, numbness, and burning or tingling sensation at limbs, Blurred vision, and Foot ulcers that refuse to heal with treatment

When diabetes is detected, common observable complications include, glaucoma, cataract formation, still births, failed marriages, neonatal deaths, and congenital defects.

Detection of diabetes, leads to the use of management approaches to conquer and control the disease condition.

Top five common management approaches to conquer diabetes include,

i.   Eating balanced Diets

The importance of consuming balanced diets cannot be overemphasized, when it comes to management of diabetes. Foods from meat group, milk group, cereals, bread, fruits, and vegetables, should be eaten. Avoid refined or white sugar.

Eat less fat and cholesterol. Do this by decreasing the intake of red meat, fatty foods, eggs, and cheese. But eat more of fish.

i.   Avoid Caffeine, Alcohol, and Smoking

These are harmful to the body, as they try to distort the body's normal functioning.

ii.   Lose Some Weight or Add Some Weight

If one is overweight, it is advisable to shed some weight. This can be done by reducing the quantity of food consumed by half or by consuming fewer calories.

For the underweight, it is advisable to add some weight, by eating diets containing enough calories with minimum sugar, to help build up body mass. With this approach, a normal weight can be maintained, which is reasonable.

iii.　　　Undertake Regular Exercise

Schedule a regular program of exercise, to help burn down sugar and control diabetes. Exercise should be done on daily basis, to be able to reap its benefits. Exercises to perform include running, walking, stretching your body, swimming, etc.

iv.　　　Get Artificially Administered Insulin Through a Doctor

Your type or dosage of insulin should be determined by your doctor, to avoid over-utilization or under-utilization, which may accompany self medication.

With the above detection and management approaches to conquer diabetes, be rest assured that diabetes shall be controlled.

vii. Combating Breast cancer

Seven Secrets Experts Reveal for Preventing Breast Cancer

B reast cancer can be prevented. It is a well known fact that breast cancer has no cure as yet, but early detection can help control it.

The following revealed secrets can help many women to prevent, detect, and control the disease:

1. Avoid Stress In Your Daily Life.

Experts say that there is a link between stress and the risk of having breast cancer. Stress lowers the body's immune system, and causes your body to become easily attacked by diseases, including breast cancer.

2. Eat Balanced Diets.

Eating balanced diets helps to build your body's immune system, keeping strong and able to resist diseases.

Your balanced diet should consist of the following types of foods to be eaten:

i. Eat a lot of natural fruits and vegetables.

They would protect your body cells from damage. You should eat up to five or more servings of fruits and vegetables daily. Eat cabbage, broccoli, cauliflower, Brussels, and apricots.

ii. Your Diet should have A High Fiber Content.

Wheat bran and beans is highly recommended.

iii. Avoid fatty Foods.

Eat low fat diets to help prevent cancer. You can daily consume one tablespoon of olive oil to reduce breast cancer risk by 50 percent.

Too much fat in your body causes obesity, which is a risk factor for breast cancer among women above 50 years of age.

iv. Avoid over processed food.

v. Consume vitamin D rich products.

vi. Take a multivitamin capsule daily.

3. Avoid Smoking And Drinking Alcohol.

These are risk behaviors you must avoid. Smoking cigarette and marijuana is very dangerous to your health.

Alcohol also is a silent killer. These are risk factors for breast cancer.

4. Have daily and regular Exercise.

Do constant deep breathing and aerobic exercises. By exercising regularly, breast cancer risk is lowered. Thus exercise prevents breast cancer.

5. Get Self Education.

Ask more questions about breast cancer, make findings about your about your family history, study these preventives measures and apply them.

6. Keep Slim And Avoid Obesity.

Check your weight and avoid being over-weight. Obesity increases breast cancer risk.

7. Do Self Breast Examination.

Regular self examination of breast would help early detection. Common detection signs are lumps, thickening, swelling, reddening or darkening of breast, scaling at nipples, etc.

It is possible to prevent breast cancer when they above measures are adopted.

CHAPTER 2

SPECIFIC HABITS REQUIRING CHANGE

There are some habits that have become part of a lifestyle, which require change in order to achieve that desired healthier and younger looking life.

i. Alcohol Addiction

Workable Steps to Quit Drinking Alcohol

Workable steps to quit drinking alcohol abound. What actually are the causes of drinking alcohol and have people involved bothered about quit measures of drinking alcohol?

Alcohol has a depressant effect on your brain when taken and the depressant effect hinders the normal functioning of the brain. Yet some people believe that it is a stimulant.

Among the effect of alcohol on the brain is the reduction in self control and judgment impairment. When your self control is diminished though alcoholic intake, you would say or do things in which you would not normally say or do.

Your judgment becomes impaired in that; you begin to take abnormal risks, liking jumping from a moving vehicle and driving in a reckless manner. You can see that victims here never took any workable steps to quit drinking, so they do what they do.

Alcohol has brought much joy to man, along with much suffering, especially to women and children of men who are drunkards.

Alcohol removes self respect and sober lifestyles, and brings about unhappiness, violence, rape, waste, and fighting, leaving the loved ones within a family most affected. Some parents drink and keep their children and family in hunger.

Alcohol induces a kind of false or fake happiness. This is done by diminishing your anxiousness, tension, stress. When this happens the person involves begins to act in a cheerful and joyful manner. This causes many people to become addicted to alcohol in order to forget their sorrows and problems, in a momentary way.

Some persons have lost their jobs, reduced their job performance, diminished their mental and physical health, divorced their wives, fallen into a ditch or gutter, have broken homes and marriages, and have become socially unfit, due to alcohol dependence for the inducement of the above mentioned fake hope.

A person may become a drunkard when he or she becomes totally dependent on alcohol, leading to unwanted behaviors. The causes of drinking alcohol are many and varied.

Though causes of alcohol are complicated, yet when an individual who is addicted or dependence on alcohol drinking, can quit if he or she so desires.

If you are willing to quit, there will be a way out for you. You can take following workable steps to quit drinking alcohol and regain your lost family relationships, and glories.

1. Eat balanced Diets

Start with eating balanced diets. Avoid sweets, fried foods, over processed foods, and too much starchy foods. Eat much of fruits and vegetables on a daily basis. Eating balanced diets will help build up your body's ability to quit drinking.

2. Take fruit juice or Snack on a Fruit when Desiring to Drink

Whenever you have the temptation or ill desire to drink, get a fruit juice or snack on a fruit.

3. Get your Spouse or co-workers Informed about your desire to quit drinking.

Your wife or husband, co-worker or any close person of yours should be notified of your intention to quit drinking.

This would enable you to make bold attempts to quit without any feeling of inferiority, and also, to be helped out of the bad habit through concentrated efforts.

4. Stop Going to Drinking Joints.

Where you are used to gathering with others to drink excessively, you must apply conscious effort to avoid such gathering, places, or joints, hotel or bar.

Inform your friends that you go along to drink and avoid them, when they call on you for drinking.

5. Consciously stop Budgeting for Alcohol Drinking

When you draw up your daily, weekly, or monthly budgets, deliberately stop budgeting for drinking. This would help you to easily quit drinking alcohol.

6. Close any Bar in your Home

If you have a drinking bar in your home, close it, and take out all drinks, bottles and drinking gadgets. Destroy them and restructure that part of your home in which you used as a bar.

7. Seek Medical Help

If you are such a chronic alcoholic, you need psychiatric help to conquer the intensity of your inward feelings and conflicts.

You can be helped with some drugs that would cause you to be sensitive to alcohol, make you ill and vomit whenever you drink. See your doctor.

8. Surrender your Life to God

When God comes to your situation, you know that all is well. So, get born-again. I mean repent of your sins, through Jesus Christ. Return to God.

You can see a true servant of God nearer you to help you, if only you are willing to quit drinking and willing to become a true Christian. This will muster Heaven's power to help you say bye to alcohol drinking.

ii. Smoking

Saying Bye to Grave Dangers of Smoking

Saying bye to grave dangers of smoking becomes possible when one acknowledges that tobacco is the most single inescapable health problem today in the world.

Records have it that tobacco is the cause of many deaths all over the world. On a yearly basis, many die mainly from cancer and heart diseases.

This is in addition to the halitosis, the stained fingers and teeth, the foul-smelling clothes, the smoker's cough, pains, and suffering.

Many health risks abound to smokers as compared to non-smokers. A smoker may say cigarette relaxes me in times of stress. Such must consider also the vulnerability of cancer of the bladder to which cigarette smoking brings.

How is it that cigarette smoking brings in such chronic sicknesses and even deaths? It happens that the respiratory tract of the lungs has lining of tiny hairs that help to flush out any mucus and foreign matter in the bronchi up to the throat, to be spit out through the mouth. Inhaling tobacco causes these little tiny hairs to become paralyzed.

But while asleep and not smoking these cilia begin to recover, all through the night they stand up pushing upward, all the junk of tobacco. In the morning that is what you cough off with the familiar smokers cough.

After smoking for years, your powerful working cilia become totally destroyed, and never able to rise up again at night to try and perform their function of throwing orb pushing up junk.

With this development, the mucus that have trapped pollutants, dust, tobacco junk, and foreign matter that you have inhaled, being accumulated, just deposits and remains there, instead of being pushed up and out.

These deposits become the breeding ground of bacteria and viruses, leading to colds, chronic bronchitis, respiratory infections, and other chronic diseases.

Smoking cigarette also brings about a disease in which the lung is less elastic, destroying the alveoli and air sacs that permit the exchange of oxygen for carbon dioxide.

Smoking causes lung cancer, in which statistics has it that eighty five percent of lung cancer cases are in men, and seventy five percent in women are connected to smoking cigarette. Cigarette smoking is a major cause of cancer death.

When a cigarette smoker inhales and drags the cigarette smoke into his or her lungs, poisonous gases and compounds, including cyanide, carbon monoxide, and volatile aromatic hydrocarbons.

The poisonous gases and compounds enter the bloodstream and go straight to the heart. Within seven seconds, the nicotine is pumped from the heart to brain, where it is absorbed, triggering the release of substances called, catecholamine, which produce adrenaline-like effect, increasing the heart rate and blood pressure. This makes smokers to feel high.

Smoking is an addiction, which though difficult to quit, need be abandoned. This will save your life the entire heart ache, heart diseases, and many other troubles.

But you can quit if you are willing. For where there is a will to quit smoking, there is certainly going to be a way to quit smoking.

iii. Drug Addiction

Danger of Drug Abuse

There is grave danger in drug addiction. Becoming addicted to drug such as marijuana, cocaine and heroin has many grave consequences, some of which are neurological disorders, behavioral and personality changes, cardiac and respiratory troubles, and death.

Do your best to avoid such dangerous drugs that poses serious threat to health and long life.

CHAPTER 3

HEALTHY LIVING

How to Have a Healthy Blood Stream without Anemia

Anemia is a blood disease, which is sometimes call ' thin blood '. There are many kinds of anemia, but the common types are iron deficiency anemia and pernicious anemia.

Sometimes anemia occurs as a result of the destruction of too many red blood cells or the loss of too many red blood cells through direct or hidden bleeding.

The more common forms of anemia are caused by a failure of the blood forming system, located at the bone marrow, to manufacture adequate or the right type of red blood cells.

This failure is usually because of the lack of iron and other essential nutrients in the diet.

Anemia symptoms include:

a) A pale skin and mucous membranes

b) Loss of appetite

c) Easy fatigue

d). Low energy

e) Shortness of breath

f) Palpitation of the heart and

g) General weakness.

In onset of pernicious anemia, symptom includes, numbness, tingling, and needles-and-pins sensations in the arms and legs. In addition the tongue may be sore and smooth.

You can enable your blood stream to begin to flow strongly and smoothly, by starting to revitalize your blood. To do this effectively, you need iron and copper.

Wheat germ, molasses, and liver are the best sources of iron and copper. Plan to begin consuming liver once or twice a week, including wheat germ and molasses without sulphur, in your day to day eating or diets.

Inadequate or unbalanced diets lacking in iron, copper, proteins, and vitamin B, results in marginal anemia, a situation where the body cannot produce enough healthy blood cells, to maintain a healthy blood stream.

Report that all ages have a common complaint about this type of anemia.

The red cells contain more protein than iron, this makes protein of necessity. You also need all the essential amino acid for the optimal building of your blood.

Women are more vulnerable to anemia condition than men, because that lose blood on a monthly basis. They therefore net properly handle the problem of anemia.

It is possible to easily correct an anemic situation or condition, when your diet contain optimal amounts of complete protein, made available through milk, meat, eggs, wheat germ and brewer's yeast.

The formation of a healthy blood must obtain all of vitamin B, namely thiamine, niacin, folic acid, etc. It is known that lack of folic acid and vitamin B12, seem to be a cause of anemic condition, called pernicious anemia.

10 Tips for Prevention of Diseases and Conditions

The need to prevent diseases and conditions cannot be overemphasized. To remain healthy, prevention must be considered.

The following tips or steps when undertaken would help in the prevention of diseases and conditions.

1. Improve Your Health Knowledge And Awareness.

If you are not informed, you become deformed. Without health literacy, you would lack knowledge; you become misinformed about the body and the causes of diseases and conditions.

Lack of knowledge makes it difficult to understand the importance of lifestyle factors like diet and exercise would make it difficult take care.

You must become aware of health conditions and diseases, and obtain knowledge about them. This would help you to prevent diseases and conditions.

2. Avoid All Known Causes Of Illness.

For example common cold is the most frequently occurring in the world, and is responsible for people absenting themselves from work and school. You must avoid the known cause of this illness.

Also, abdominal pain, diarrhea, and vomiting are mostly caused by food poisoning. So, avoid the means of food poisoning. Check and do so for other diseases and conditions.

3. Avoid Contracting HIV/AIDS.

To avoid contracting and contacting HIV/AIDS, take the following measures:

a. Get married if still single.

b. Have sex with your wife only and avoid multiple sex partners.

c. Practice abstinence if you are still single.

d. Say No to sex outside marriage or avoid premarital sex.

e. Avoid direct contact with blood.

f. Do not share needles or sharp objects like blades with other people.

g. Avoid transfusing unscreened blood.

4. Avoid Accidents And Other Hazards In Life.

To avoid accidents and other hazards in life, observe the following tips:

a. If you drink, do not drive.

b. Avoid eating while driving.

c. Avoid smoking while driving.

d. Avoid using cell phone while driving.

e. Put your vehicle in good condition before entering the road.

f. Observe all traffic regulations.

g. Do not walk on the left side of road facing oncoming traffic.

h. Remove sharp objects from your environment and home, example, broken bottles.

i. Stay clear from accident causing lifestyle or environments.

5. Avoid Or Quit Smoking.

Smoking is dangerous to your health and smokers are liable to die young.

Smoking of cigarette and marijuana is known to cause lung cancer, etc.

Smoking stains the teeth and gives the teeth a yellowish color.

Smoking also, causes tartar to form on the teeth.

6. Avoid Drinking Alcohol.

Alcohol causes dehydration of the body and eyes. It also causes optic nerve disease.

7. Live within a manageable stress level

Stress breaks down your immune system and makes your body vulnerable to disease attack. Limit or get rid of stress.

8. Eat Fruits and vegetables.

Eat moderate balanced diets, which must include the consumption of fruits and vegetables. Eat dark, green leafy vegetables.

Take Multivitamin Capsule Daily. This would provide all the necessary vitamins and minerals that may be missing in your diets

9. Observe Regular Daily exercise.

Exercise would keep you fresh and younger looking. Exercise enables your body to fight against diseases.

10. Get Medical Checkups And Help.

Go for medical and dental checkups every six months or once a year. Take appropriate vaccines and immunizations to strengthen your body system.

With the above tips, diseases and conditions shall be prevented and controlled, leaving you healthy looking, good, and happy.

How to Look Good through Personal Hygiene

When your personal hygiene is right, you become looking good, clean, healthy, and happy.

The following steps would help you achieve the best in this respect:

1. Observe Regular and Daily Tooth brushing.

Tooth brushing should start first thing in the morning. Brush your teeth two or three times daily, or after each meal.

Your tongue should be cleansed using your toothbrush. You must floss daily. There is the need also to see your dentist once a year.

2. Shower Twice Daily.

To look good and clean, you should shower twice daily, in the morning and at evening or night. If you involve in sports, sweat generating exercise, and in much dirty work, you need to shower at anytime you finish accomplishing such. Showering regularly helps keep away body odor.

Do not share your bathing towel. Use cotton swab to clean out excess wax in your ears.

Wash your face daily. Do so at least once a day, to remove all dirt that you may contact. This would also help keep wrinkles and pimples away.

Use a moisturizer to ensure that your face remains fresh and renewed.

3. Wash and Iron Your Clothes.

Wash your clothes after one or two times of wearing. Preferably when you sweat or notice your collar and some other parts become dirty. Ironing should also be carried out after washing and drying.

4. Keep Your Nails Trimmed.

Watch out and trim your nails when they grow. This would prevent debris or dirt underneath the nails.

5. Remove Unwanted Hair.

To look gook and clean, you need to get rid of unwanted hair on your face or other places you do not want them to appear.

Remove hair that grow out of your nostrils, ears, chin, upper and lower lips, etc. you can shave or use any other hair removal strategy, like hot waxing, laser hair removal, and electrolysis method, etc.

Have the hair on your head cut if grown. This is determined by the length of your hair. You can get your hair cut in every six to ten weeks.

Keep the hair on your head clean and conditioned, to enable it become strong and healthy. Do not wash it too frequently, to avoid making it dry and brittle.

6. Use Acne Prevention Cleanser.

If you have acne, use acne prevention cleanser to cover breakouts and prevent further acne. Do not squeeze or pick on the acne, this would worsen the situation.

Use oil blotting sheets for oily skin. Get the blotting sheets and soak out oil from your face throughout the day. This would enable your face look good and clean.

7. Care for Your Feet to Avoid Foot Troubles and Odor.

Sun dry shoes due to sweat or air out your shoes after wearing, and change socks. Dust your shoes with baby powder. Do not wear shoes without socks, to avoid odor.

Dress cuts and burns if present. Cover all cuts, sores, and burns regularly. Better prevent yourself from having cuts and burns.

8. Avoid Strong Fragrance Or Perfumes.

Use soaps with less fragrance, which may cause offensive odor. Shower with less harsh or gentle soap.

Also, perfumes with strong fragrance, which produces strong and offensive odor, should be avoided. Maintain a clean personal hygiene, and there would be no need of perfumes.

9. Observe Regular Washing Of Hands.

Most infections are got through the hands. So, wash your hands often to keep germs away.

Wash your hands with soap after touching saliva or vomit, after contact with animals, rubbish bins, the sick, after work, or after changing infants diaper, etc.

With the above tips for personal hygiene, you shall become good looking and clean.

Environment and Your Health

Environmental pollution is dangerous to your health, because what happens outside would definitely affect what happens inside your body.

Harmful emissions from vehicles, generators, and other machines giving out fumes from their exhaust, go along way in affecting your environment.

Also, industrial and agricultural firms dump their wastes which are contaminants to our environment. Some of these contaminants are deposited in our open waters.

Smoke from exhaust and smokers are harmful to the body when inhaled, because it is made up of a harmful gas called carbon monoxide.

Automobile emissions add up to the build up of carbon dioxide. This becomes a problem when the volume becomes more than what is needed.

Your health can be affected greatly by the accumulation of these pollutants, leading to cancer and other infectious diseases.

In some places, human waste which is used for fertilizer contains toxins. When these toxins are absorbed by plants and we eat the plants, health problems may arise. Water can be contaminated with medicines from many patients, like hepatitis patients.

In addition, toxic waste from feces goes along way to affect one's health, if such water is consumed.

Pesticides and fertilizer residues from both are water and food, becomes dangerous when taken in. In some cosmetics and medicines, toxins additives and other substances are dangerous to your health.

Many are unaware of the harmful effects of caffeine that is being consumed daily by many. Also, Cigarette and marijuana are dangerous producers of harmful smoke that may affect the body. Sulfur and nitrogen oxides from coal burning equipment and factories, get combined in the atmosphere and drop as rain, snow, and dust. This leads to environmental destruction which may affect your health.

The use of pesticides and chemical fertilizers made up of nitrogen, phosphorus, and potassium, produces nitrates from runoffs or irrigation, which end up in rivers, ponds, and wells, leading to water contamination. This makes the water unfit for human and animal consumption.

Most processed foods have a higher concentration of pesticides. This is harmful to your health. Also, food coloring and preservatives that are used for most processed foods are dangerous to your health.

Environmental pollution has penetrated indoors, sending in toxins, such as benzene, formaldehyde, and chloroform. In trying to keep the home in an air tight condition, pollution arises. This is just sealing of us with pollutants which are dangerous to health. Formaldehyde is known to cause headache, eye irritation, depression, and asthma.

We cannot live without air. We need oxygen for our survival. The oxygen we take in enters our blood system, and is being transported to various cells of the body, to generate energy for our livelihood.

As such we need to take care of the air we breathe and our general environment. This would go along way to keeps our body healthy and free from the various harmful effects of environmental pollution.

So, watch your environment, and make sure that the various toxins, and pollutants, that many have been caught up with, do not have an entrance into your body. By this you would be free.

Health Benefits of Increasing Your Fiber Consumption

Fibers are a group of complex carbohydrates, with no nutritive value because of their non-digestive nature. They include cellulose, vegetable gums and pectin.

They are important in a healthy diet. The human body has no enzymes that are able to break down fiber.

So, they are therefore not digested when consumed, but passes through from the mouth to the intestines, and end up as part of the bulk of feces, which then is passed out of the body.

We have two fiber types, the soluble and non-soluble. Soluble fibers are present in dried beans, peanuts, apple, barley, oat bran, strawberries, and oat meal.

These soluble fibers have been found to reduce or lower high cholesterol and triglycerides and helps control the level of sugar in the blood.

This is done by the fiber being able to deal with cholesterol in the intestines and sending it out of the body.

Non-soluble fibers are found in wheat bran, fruits, vegetables, whole grain, breads, and cereals. They are known to help in controlling diarrhea, constipation, diverticulitis, and hemorrhoids.

Your body would work well when provided with both soluble and non-soluble fibers. The soluble fiber enables the stool to be bulky and soft, and the non-soluble drives it along.

These fibers need water to enable their proper functioning. As such it is recommended that you drink 8-10 glasses of water daily, and a glass of water be taken before and after meal, and not with the meal.

Researchers say that soluble fiber is important in glucose control and recommends fiber foods such as oranges, grapefruits, oatmeal, oat bran, papayas, Lima beans, raisins, prunes, zucchini, cantaloupes, and low-fat granola.

Though fiber is indigestible, fiber has been found to have many benefits of which some are stated above, thus: Fiber has been found to lower blood pressure.

Fiber has been found to protect against heart disease by being able to lower the bad cholesterol level in your body. Fiber provides a bulky mass in the intestines and therefore reduces hunger pangs by keeping you full.

Increased fiber intake has been found to help in a low incidence of many kinds of cancers, especially colon cancer.

Fiber is known to fight against disease due to its ability to regulate the gastrointestinal tract. It also helps to keep the energy levels at balance.

You need to increase or double your fiber intake to be able to reap the various benefits of fiber, by making use of whole grains such as brown rice, oats, and whole wheat (100 percent whole wheat).

Consume fruits and vegetables with their skins on after washing. Eat more of raw and lightly cooked vegetables in the non-processed state, to avoid reducing the fiber effectiveness.

Also, increase your intake of raw oat bran from oat meal and wheat bran.

10 Secrets for Whiter and Brighter Teeth

The top 10 secrets for having a whiter and brighter teeth, gives all that you need to achieve or experience a whiter and brighter teeth.

You should start seeing the difference, as you get through the following 10 secrets for having whiter and brighter teeth:

1. Have A Good Toothbrush.

Toothbrush is the most common device that is used for removal of plaque and the maintenance of healthy whiter teeth.

Many factors are to be taken into consideration when selecting a toothbrush. You must start with purchasing a good toothbrush with firm bristles that are soft nylon to avoid scratching your gums.

Such brush should be easily handled and able to remove tartar or plaques without giving you injury.

The bristles of your brush should be soft and such brush should be able to reach every tooth in your mouth.

Toothbrush replacement should be done every three months, when the bristles are worn out and after an illness.

Electric brushes can be used also, especially for children and the handicaps.

2. Observe Regular and Proper Tooth Brushing

To prevent plaque forming and stains setting in, it is advisable to brush your teeth twice a day, early in the morning after your breakfast and last thing before you go to bed or every 12 hours and after every meal.

You can brush gently, up and down, at a circular or 45 degree angle. Do brush inside the teeth also.

Regular tooth-brushing with or without a toothpaste, would help in avoiding plaque or tooth loss and offer you a good oral hygiene maintenance.

3. Observe A Regular Teeth Flossing Habit.

Teeth's flossing is an essential part of cleaning your teeth. Flossing helps to remove plaque between teeth and at gum area. You can see your dentist to help you do this better.

Without flossing, your teeth can never be totally clean. This should be done once a day to remove stains that try to form between teeth.

4. Cleanse Your Teeth Through A Dentist.

To have cleaner teeth, have a dentist cleanse your teeth once a year. In general whitening your teeth at home is quite cheaper than contacting a professional.

5. Avoid Red wine And Coffee.

Red wine and coffee are known to stain the teeth very fast, so keep away from them.

6. Make use Of Baking Soda and Hydrogen Peroxide.

You can use baking soda with hydrogen peroxide added, to make a paste, for your teeth brushing three times a day. This would help you have whiter teeth.

7. Avoid or Stop Smoking.

In order not to have yellow teeth and sometimes burnt teeth, stay free from smoking of cigarette.

8. Use of Lemon Massage and Lemon Juice Mouthwash.

Make use of lemon peel to massage your teeth and rinse, to whiten your teeth. Also, lemon juice with hot water as mouthwash can be used to remove tartar.

9. Use of Salt for Brushing.

The use of salt to brush the teeth from time to time whitens the teeth and firms the gums. Also, for perfect white teeth, mix salt with lime juice and clean your teeth.

10.   Make use of Raw Vegetables, Banana Peel and Strawberries

Raw vegetables have a natural cleansing power, use them.

Trying out or maintaining the above revealed secrets of teeth whitening on a regular or daily basis would help you achieve a healthier, whiter, and brighter teeth, that can also enable you to always put up a confident and charming smile.

Vitamin C: Cancer Destroyer and Immune System Booster

Research continue to show that a combination of environmental toxins including tobacco, poor diet and lifestyle issues contribute significantly to the incidence of cancer in our society today.

While a poor diet may certainly increase cancer risk, importantly, a good diet may also lower cancer risk.

This probably is the reason why American Cancer Society recommends the eating of plenty of vitamin C-rich fruits and vegetables.

Recently published research has stated that a high dose of intravenous vitamin C may be effective in treating cancer. Those studies in the 1970s first made a suggestion that when high doses of Vitamin C are given, may bring about some benefits clinically, but later studies proved it wrong.

Researchers now say that the same result could not be gotten because the original studies used both intravenous and oral administration, while later studies used only oral administration. Thus the differences might have given the disparity.

Normalizing your vitamin C intake can bring about the boosting of your immune system to fight against unwanted viruses, bacteria, and other toxins. Vitamin C acts synergistically, by working with other nutrients including flavornoids, carotenoids, vitamin E, and many minerals to build up your body's defense against diseases.

Higher than RDA intakes of vitamin C enhances the effective functioning of your blood and cardiovascular system by boosting the good cholesterol, lowering blood pressure, and lowering bad cholestcrol.

Environmental pollutants and smoke from cigarettes depletes vitamin C. As such The US National Academy of Sciences recommends that smokers and non-smokers should almost double the dose intake of vitamin C. It has been stated by experts that vitamin c has antihistamine effects that has been shown, help improve airflow and improve respiratory measurements.

Vitamin c is more concentrated in the lens tissue than in the blood. This is an indication of how necessary vitamin C is in bringing about visual health.

Low optimal vitamin C levels contribute to muscle weakness and soreness, bringing about a decreased ability to utilize fatty acids and can compromise the body's ability to heal from injuries among other things.

Use of Vitamin C supplements helps healing of wounds and reduces stress experienced during exercise.

Vitamin C is necessary in building and maintaining well-developed blood vessels and gums.

It also helps to prevent infections. A diet lacking in fresh fruits and vegetables results in a disease called scurvy – swelling of the tongue and bleeding of the gums and joints.

The best sources of vitamin C are all the citrus fruits (orange, lime, lemon, grapefruit, and tangerine), tomatoes, green peppers, cabbage, and uncooked leafy vegetables such as lettuce.

Oxygen destroys vitamin C, while canning and freezing preserves some vitamin C.

Recommended daily serving of vitamin C is 4 – 5 servings of fresh fruits and vegetables. This would enable you to enjoy all the benefits that the vitamin gives.

Foods and Supplements to Prevent and Improve Poor Eyesight

Your eyes respond to lifestyle and dietary changes, which may go along way to promote healthy eyesight or bring about poor eyesight.

Foods and supplements have a role to play in preventing and improving poor eyesight.

As one continues to age, the eyes become less active, but foods and supplements can be used to prevent or improve them.

As you age, old sightedness, a type of farsighted that results from aging occurs. This type of farsightedness comes normally and gradually with age.

With age, the crystalline lens of the eyes becomes less transparent, and tends to lose its elasticity.

The lens at this time fails to thicken properly and casts images behind instead of on the retina. Some persons at the age of forty and above begin to hold the newspaper farther and farther away, to be able to read it.

Damage to the eyes is often caused by environmental pollution, toxins, and poor diets deficient in essential nutrients.

Damage is also caused by bye products of normal functioning of the body. Eye diseases such as cataracts, glaucoma, and age-related eye degeneration, may occur as from age 40 and above.

Foods and supplements can help prevent and improve poor eyesight, because the eyes respond well to lifestyle changes and diets.

The following foods and supplements can help prevent and improve poor eyesight:

1. Eat Garlic and onions

These foods contain sulphur, which form glutathione. Glutathione protects the lens, and aids in the prevention of cataracts, experts say.

2. Add Bilberry to your Diet

This food helps strengthen capillaries in the eyes, improves blood circulation to the retina, and helps the production of a purple pigment that is used by the eye rods for night vision, experts say.

3. Eat Red Peppers and Tomatoes

These foods are also known to reduce the risk of cataracts. These foods contain good amounts of vitamin C.

4. Eat Yellow Vegetables, Carrot and deep Oranges

They contain beta-carotene, which help to reduce the risk of eye degeneration trouble due to age.

5. Eat Broccoli, Spinach, and Green vegetables

Experts say that they help to shield the eyes from ultra violet rays.

6. Daily Ingest Multivitamins and Antioxidants Supplements

You must daily take antioxidants and multivitamins supplements. These provide all the essential nutrients that are required by the eye for normal and optimal functioning, which may be missing in your diets. They will aid the eye to receive normal blood circulation, nerve function, and general eye health.

Necessity of Vitamins and Supplements for Healthy Living

Vitamins are organic substances produced from plants and some animal sources. For an individual to remain healthy and grow normally, vitamins are required in very small quantities.

Lack of the necessary amounts, however small may bring about a vitamin deficiency disease, called a vitaminosis. Examples of such diseases include beriberi, rickets, scurvy, and pellagra.

Vitamin supplements are sometimes clearly necessary, whenever the dietary intake of vitamins is inadequate. Multivitamins plus minerals in capsule or tablet form, taken once a day goes along way to fortify your diet. However, a good mixed diet of common foods, supplies all the vitamins you need.

But because a good mixed diet of common foods, including protective foods, may be lacking, or if present, may be destroyed through cooking, there is therefore the need for a multivitamins plus minerals capsule or tablets to be taken daily. Sometimes this problem occurs when on a low-calorie reducing diet, after surgical operation, during pregnancy, and during a serious illness.

Vitamin deficiency are mostly of multiple rather than single in a particular diet, it is therefore necessary to take vitamin supplements prescribed to treat certain diseases and conditions, because, they supply a balance of all vitamins.

It is now recommended that a mixed diet should be taken, so that all the vitamins will be present. In considering a mixed diet, only a few vitamins should be taken seriously. This is so because, when these few vitamins are present, others also become present. These vitamins of importance are vitamin A, C, D, and three members of vitamin B complex (thiamine, niacin, and riboflavin).

Vitamin A (retinol)

Vitamin A is essential to growth and development. It maintains the normal functioning of the cells lining the throat and the eyelids. It is needed for normal night vision.

Vitamin A aids growth and tooth formation. If absent or deficient, or lacking, results in night blindness- seeing poorly in the dim light.

It reduces resistance to colds and other throat and eye infections. Continued shortage of vitamin A may result in blindness.

Sources of vitamin A are liver, kidneys, whole milk, butter, eggs, and tomatoes, all green and yellow vegetables (carrots, corn, and sweet potatoes).

These yellow vegetables contain carotene, a substance from which vitamin A is produced. Palm oil is very rich in carotene. A mixed diet containing the above sources is very necessary for good health.

Vitamin B complex comprises of a large number of water soluble vitamins, including thiamine, riboflavin, niacin, folic acid, etc.

Thiamine is essential for utilization of carbohydrates, normal appetite, and function of the digestive tract. Severe deficiency results in beriberi- a serious nervous disorder.

Sources of thiamine are whole grains, meat, fish, and vegetables. Proper cooking is required in order not to destroy it.

Riboflavin is essential for growth, health, and cell respiration. It helps to maintain healthy skin and proper coordination of muscles. Deficiency results in stunted growth, scaly, sore skin and eye diseases.

The vitamin is found in yeast, liver, kidneys, milk, eggs, and green vegetables. Niacin is needed for proper use of carbohydrates in the body. It is also called pellagra-preventive vitamin.

Deficiency results in skin rash, stomach upset, paralysis and mental disorders. Sources are garden vegetables, lean meat, liver, eggs, and yeast.

Vitamin C (ascorbic acid)

This vitamin is necessary in building and maintaining well-developed blood vessels and gums. It also helps to prevent infections.

Deficiency causes blood vessels to break down, and a serious disease called scurvy develops (swelling of the tongues and bleeding of the gums and joints).

Best sources are all the citrus fruits (orange, lime, lemon, grapefruit, and tangerine), tomatoes, green peppers, cabbage, and uncooked leafy vegetables such as lettuce.

Vitamin D (calciferol)

Vitamin D is also called the Sunshine Vitamin. It can be manufactured in the skin. Lack of this vitamin D in the body can result in rickets (faulty growth of bones and teeth in children).

This may cause deformed chest and bow legs. Sources found are liver, fish liver oil, milk, and eggs.

It is better to fortify your diet with a multiple vitamins plus minerals capsule or tablets, in case the inability to provide a mixed diet containing all the vitamins and minerals or should some be destroyed through cooking.

The best way to Handle and Cure Food Poisoning

Food poisoning may be classified as an accident case or disease condition. Salmonella is the germ or microbe that causes the problem, but other germs are sometimes responsible.

Viruses, bacteria, and other microbes found in foods which were improperly taken care of, not stored in the fridge when not in use, and in undercooked foods, are causative agents.

Usually, the stomach is the point of trouble. Symptoms of severe intestinal infection are diarrhea, vomiting, nausea, and abdominal pains.

The most dangerous, severe and fatal type of food poisoning is called botulism. It's caused by a microbe called clostridium botullinus.

This type of poison is one of the most troublesome and most fatal. Its additional symptoms include difficulty in seeing and double vision.

The best way to handle and cure food poisoning is to follow the steps below:

1. Take Much Fluid to Remain Hydrated

Drink enough water and fruit juices, avoiding the citrus fruit juice, which can irritate the stomach. One or two teaspoons of powdered mustard water in a glass of slightly warm water.

This should be repeated in 15 minutes time, should more fluid is being needed.

2. Take Activated Charcoal

For a period of about one hour, take 6 to 7 capsules of activated charcoal.

A powder that is also used consists of two parts of activated charcoal, and one part each of magnesium oxide and tannic acid.

The charcoal would help to bind the microbes causing the problem in the intestines, making it possible for their easy elimination. This action would bring about freedom or less severe pains or attack.

3. Give about 2 or 3 glassful, of either warm or cold milk

4. Take herbal remedy to boost immunity.

Take 3/4 teaspoon of Golden seal extract (Hydrastis canadensis) and Echinacea spp in half cup of water can be taken to strengthen your immune system, and also fight the microbes in charge.

5. Seek Medical Assistance

If the symptoms still persist in the face of taking antidotes, after two days, consult your doctor.

It is very important for you to prevent accidental or disease attacks due to food poisoning, making sure that foods tasting and smelling differently be avoided or discarded.

Secrets of Keeping Away Sicknesses through Washing of Hands

It is very important to wash your hands on a regular basis. The following secrets would help you become free from certain sicknesses:

1. How Washing Of Hands Prevent Sicknesses.

By washing your hands regularly, you keep away germs that have been picked up from the environment, people, places, toilet, animals, and the air.

When you pick these germs, it is easy to use your hands, to rub your nose and eyes, and even put into your mouth. Thus, with contaminated hands, you become contaminated and get a sickness.

Sicknesses such common colds, hepatitis A, meningitis, and infectious diarrhea, can be prevented, if you form the habit of regular washing of hands.

2. Cultivate A Regular Habit of Washing Your Hands.

Practice washing your hands when you do the following activities:

i). When your hands look dirty.

ii). when you handle animals and enter their housing.

iii). Wash before you prepare food.

iv). Wash food preparation time

v). Wash after food preparation.

vi). Wash before eating your meals.

vii). Wash after eating your meals.

viii).wash after using toilet or urinary.

ix). Wash after handling patients or sick persons.

x). Wash after retuning from garden or any other work.

xi). Wash after doing nothing and using the rest room.

xii). Wash your hands when they touch saliva or vomit.

xiii). Wash after handling garbage.

xiv). Wash your hands after sneezing, coughing or blowing your nose.

3. Observe Best Hand Washing Procedures.

When you become conscious of the need to wash your hands to avoid germs, adopt the following procedures:

i. Wet your hands with clean water.

ii. Apply bar or liquid soap.

ii. Wash your hands by rubbing and scrubbing your hands together.

iii. Scrub the surfaces of your hands.

iv. Wash for about 30 seconds or if heavily soiled, till they look clean.

v. Rinse your hands and dry them with a clean towel.

4. Care for Your Towels and Handkerchief.

With heavy use, towels and handkerchiefs carry germs. For the ones that are heavily used, change them daily, practice hanging them up to dry, to reduce the risk of contacting germs. Wash regularly. Preferably, you can use paper towels.

5. Always Use A Hand Lotion After Washing Hands.

Too much of hand washing can cause your hands to become dry and develop chapped skin on hands, which can crack and give way for germs to enter.

So, use a hand lotion to avoid these, and make your hands look soft, smooth, and good looking.

The above suggestions can help you to have good health. Following and practicing them regularly, would also save a lot of money that would have been given to drugstores and medical professionals.

CHAPTER 4

YOUR SKIN AND LOOKING YOUNGER

Beauty and Immunity Boosting Foods That Fight Aging

S ome beauty foods and immunity boosting foods that fight wrinkles smooth the skin, give healthy eyes, and drives cold and flu.

Eating special foods is a must for those who want to look younger and beautiful. When looking for such foods, beauty and immunity boosting foods should come readily in mind.

The following beauty foods are also able to build up the muscles and burn of fats in the body:

1. Sweet potatoes - Smoothes your skin

This vegetable is packed full with beauty boosting anti oxidant, called beta carotene. When you consume sweet potatoes, your body works on the beta carotene and convert it to vitamin A, which then keeps your skin to be silky smooth.

A serving of sweet potatoes provides a double dose of vitamin A needs and has more than 10,000mg of beta carotene, which researchers say is linked to sun damage protection.

2. Blueberries - Fights wrinkles

The garnish, blueberries, in your morning oatmeal, can help to lower the signs of aging, with high antioxidant content, vitamin C and E in particular, which strengthens collagen formation by reducing harmful free radical damage.

Report has it that researches at the United States Department of Agriculture (USDA) have found that a serving of blueberries gives the most antioxidants when compared to other fruits and vegetables.

It is recommended that you blend it and toss half a cup of blueberries into your shakes.

3. Spinach - gives good eye health

It is reported that most people depended on spinach for muscle strength, and that eating spinach is a major reason why many people do not need eyeglasses.

Also, according to USDA, spinach properties are known for prevent vision loss among vegetables.

Experts say that boosting your daily diet with foods, such as spinach, may help save your eyesight if you stay all day in front of your computer.

It is recommended that you add olive oil, garlic, and lemon juice, and cook for two minutes.

4. Mushrooms

It is recommended that you toss in mushrooms. Mushrooms, according to research, are said to contain a type of sugar, has potent antiviral and antibacterial properties.

5. Salmon

It is reported that salmon contain lean protein that fights diseases, and also has good fats that help strengthen cell membranes, which help to speed up any healing time.

6. Pumpkin and other Leafy vegetables

These vegetables contain photochemical plant compounds that fight disease-causing free radicals.

7. Garlic

Garlic is a natural germ fighter. It is made up of an antibacterial compound. Research has it that this helps to stimulate white blood cells involved in immunity work. It is recommended that you take two raw gloves of garlic daily.

Ways to Restore Your Skin to Perfect Beauty

In looking good through attaining and maintaining a beautiful skin, you need to put in effort to achieve this feat by following the under listed ways, to restore your skin to perfect beauty.

1. Use Moisturizing Soaks to Soothe Dryness

Get a winter sunflower bath by compounding ¼ cup shelled, unsalted sunflower seed; ½ teaspoon ground cinnamon; ¼ teaspoon ground nutmeg; and ½ teaspoon vitamin E oil.

Make a fine powder of sunflower seeds and oatmeal in a food processor, add the spices and oil.

Add ¼ cup of mixture in your bath and soak for at least 20 minutes. This will help soothe, soften, and moisturize dry skin.

2. Treat Your dry Skin with Honey

Honey can be used as a natural oil free moisturizer. It pulls and attaches water to the skin. In dry or combination complexions, mix two tablespoonfuls with two teaspoon of water, and massage into your face for three minutes, then rinse.

If you have oily skin, blend a tablespoon each of honey and lemon juice, leave on skin for three minutes and rinse. For a gentle facial scrub, mix equal parts of honey and cooked oatmeal.

3. Avoid Picking at pimples if they Appear

You must avoid the temptation to pick or squeeze at your pimples if you have them. This action can cause the spread of bacteria and further infect the pore, leading to scarring.

4.   Avoid Using Hot Water on Your Face

Hot water affects the face negatively, by removing the natural oils that retain moisture and protect your skin. It also brings about conditions that require gentle care, such as inflamed capillaries and rosacea.

You can use facial cleansers with lukewarm water, two times a day. Avoid over washing your face to avoid skin sensitivity.

5.   Contact a Dermatologist for help

To avoid break outs that become much harder to cure, you need to see a dermatologist. You may be given oral prescription drugs and topical creams to control pimples and blackheads.

Seeing a dermatologist can also help you to know exactly what your condition is and avoid mistreatments that may worsen your skin condition.

Pamper your skin with a good lotion and the above ways to restore your skin to perfect beauty, and you shall look good.

Nine Ways to Prevent and Get Rid of Wrinkles

Where wrinkles are present, there is the likelihood of one's skin having that aging appearance. But for this problem you can overcome by applying the necessary measures or ways that would help eliminate and prevent wrinkles.

Given below therefore are the ways to help clear and prevent this condition.

1. Use natural facial Lotions and Creams.

These must be free from additives that can contribute to skin aging. Get and make use of keratin containing ingredients, example, cynergy TK.

This would supplement your skin naturally with keratin, to help your skin produce its own collagen and elastin - for a smooth wrinkle free skin.

Use skin care products that contain natural ingredients like Aloe Vera, collagen, glycerin, etc. Always use sunscreen creams when going outdoors.

2. Apply Honey And Lemon Juice Mask.

This should be done twice a week, and allowed for 30 minutes before washing off with water. This homemade product would brighten, soften, and improve your skin's elasticity. Thus, preventing and getting rid of wrinkles.

3. Clean Face With Milk Cream.

Do not use soap; instead clean your face with milk cream. Use moisturizing cream at night.

Mix and use egg white, one spoonful of honey and one quarter teaspoon of carrot. Apply this to the face, 30 minutes before shower in the morning, and remove after 30 minutes, with cotton wool soaked in warm water (soda bicarbonate added). This would help remove roughness and wrinkles.

4. Undertake Facial Exercises Daily.

Facial exercises would help tone the muscles of your face and get rid of wrinkles fast.

Every morning, make use of the tips of your fingers to scrub your face in upward strokes or movement.

Also, give 40 gentle taps with the tips of two fingers simultaneously placed under the two eyes. Keep your weight and do not remain thin. Remaining thin and dry encourages wrinkles.

5. Avoid Habitual Facial Expressions.

Relax your face. A tense face brings wrinkles. Avoid facial expressions like frowning and twisting the face.

6. Avoid Stress And Sleep Well.

Stress changes your body's normal functioning, and brings about aging.

7. Avoid Exposure To Sun And Heat.

Sun and heat dehydrates the skin and causes forced aging. Wear protective mask when staying near heat. Constant exposure to ultraviolet light from the sun can damage the eyes and skin, resulting in wrinkles.

8. Eat Balanced Diets.

Eat fruits and green leafy vegetables. They are filled with essential antioxidants and nutrients. Drink lots of water daily. Drink hot water with a half of lemon juice, to help flush any impurities. Take a multivitamin capsule daily. Avoid caffeine Intake.

9. Avoid Smoking And Drinking of Alcohol.

Smoking and alcohol dehydrates the skin. Smoking irritates the eyes, and brings about wrinkles.

With the above tips, you can say bye to wrinkles.

10 Steps to Get Rid of Facial Spots and Pimples

Pimples and facial spots are annoying inflammatory reactions due to the production of certain acids caused by abnormal response of some hormones circulating in the blood.

This leads to an increase production of sebum (an oily substance). Facial spots do not only affect youths, but can hang on to about 50 years of age.

To get rid of facial spots and pimples, steps or tips can help:

1. Drink More Water Daily.

Water would help to free the hair roots of the clogging oil and thus reduce oil on the face or skin. So, drink a lot of water daily, up to about two liters. Do this and your face would clear within weeks.

2. Avoid A Stressful life.

Stress causes over activity of the body chemicals or hormones, which result in facial pimples and spots.

3. Avoid Junk Foods.

Avoid fried foods, cake, sweets, pastries, and too much chocolate. They cause pimples and facial spots to form and continue. Get a chocolate free diet.

4. Live In Ventilated Rooms With Fresh Air.

Fresh air is good for your skin. Get fresh air indoors and outdoors.

5. Eat Balanced Diets.

Eat meat, eggs, fish, cheese, milk, fruits and vegetables. They would keep your skin rejuvenated.

6. Put A Face Mask Weekly.

Research the one that is best for you. For facial spots, apply lemon juice with cotton bud, to fight against bacteria.

7. Do Not Touch Or Pick Your Spots and Pimples.

Picking on spots and pimples, causes them to spread. So, do not squeeze the spots, do not cover with make-ups, and do not touch with your fingers.

8. Avoid Worry And Anxiety.

Worry aggravates the pimples and spots. Just concentrate on good things, and they shall surely clear away.

9. Get Plenty Of Rest And Sleep.

Sleep for eight hours daily, and give your body the needed rest.

10. Do Regular Face Washing.

Wash your face with water and mild soap for about two to four times a day or every three hours. Do not use sponge.

Following the above cures brings relief and clears your face of the pimples and facial spots.

Proper Eating and Best Foods for Energy

Food is the fuel of our body craves and eating the right type of food is very important, in order that we may keep our body strong and full of energy.

If you desire to loss weight, eating small amount of food, exercise regularly can be help you to achieve the goal, in addition to other things.

The following guide will help you get the best out of proper eating and best energy foods.

1. Consume the right type of food

Consume grains, fruits, and vegetables regularly. Also, make sure that you stay away from fried foods or fatty foods. Consume up to four or five small meals, rather than one or two large bowls. Try not to miss or skip breakfast or other meals, so that your body system will function normally. Avoid junk foods, like cakes, sweets, and fast foods.

2. Eat high energy foods daily to keep you on the go.

Your stress level can be managed or reduced with regular and daily consumption of high energy foods. The following best high energy foods.

a.   Oatmeal

Oatmeal is a source of fiber. Fiber has the ability to help your digestion, so that you body can have a steady flow of energy as carbohydrate enters into your blood system. Eating fiber means eating the right type of food.

b.   Beans

Beans aid the problem of low iron deficiency which brings the problem of sluggishness. Best is best eaten when prepared as soup.

c.   Snack Banana

Bananas contain potassium, a mineral element that helps in nerves and muscles normal functioning.

d. Green Spinach

Green spinach contains the magnesium mineral. Consuming spinach ensures that are taking in adequate levels of the mineral.

e. Strawberries

Strawberries can aid your body to absorb iron, because it contains vitamin C.

f. Soybean Products

Soybeans have many health benefits and contain calcium. It can be consume as soymilk, and other products.

g. Other high energy foods include tuna, whole grain bagels, and low-fat yogurt.

3. Drink water Daily and regularly

Water is very important for our body's well-being. Water helps in digestion of food in the body, and keeps the body and skin in optimal conditions.

It is recommended that you take eight to ten glasses of water daily. You can start with 2 glasses of water, first thing in the morning.

Work out your proper eating and use of best foods for energy, for good health and a better skin.

Simple Steps to Look 20 Years Younger

It is easy to look up to 20 years younger and more beautiful in six months and friends are sure to sit up and take note, if you take conscious effort and follow the outlined guide below.

The following simple steps to look 20 years younger, would aid you achieve this goal.

1. Boost your Energy

You energy level may be low, and this makes it impossible to face simple daily challenges that may confront you.

When your energy level is low, your energy drops. In order to boost your energy level, you have to ensure that you do everything possible to keep afloat.

2. Daily Observe Natural Deep Breathing and Breath properly Daily

Make sure that you take adequate amounts of fresh air daily and perform natural deep breathing exercise.

Natural deep breathing exercise can be done by breathing from your lower abdomen, inhaling slowly until your lungs are fully expanded, and then exhaling slowly after the count of ten, with your mouth open.

This will enable you to take in enough of fresh air, which is in turn supplied to all your body cells to help you look 20 years younger.

3.   Have Siesta and Catnaps for Five Minutes Daily

You must have a daily siesta of about one hour, to enable you refresh your brain and energy. In addition to a one hour daily siesta, add a five minutes catnap, to enable you get refreshed at all times.

4. Shed Excess weight

Over-weight is the cause of many health problems; therefore make sure that you cut down your weight if you have excess weight or if you are obese. Obesity can cause you diabetes and other problems.

5. Restore muscle Tone Through Physical Exercise

Physical exercise is very important. So, you must engage in daily and regular exercise. You can exercise for 30 o 60 minutes daily, indoors and outdoors.

You can do walking, jogging, swimming, dancing, bicycle riding, stretching of your body, facial exercise, etc. daily. This will tone your muscles help you look 20 years younger.

6. Eat Balanced Diets

Eating balanced diets on a daily basis would ensure that you have a complete supply of all nutrients, vitamins and minerals.

Make sure you get adequate vitamins and minerals by eating whole grains, fish instead of meat, peanut, almonds, cashew nuts, fruits and vegetables, daily.

Do not skip breakfast, because breakfast would help boost your energy from start, by providing all the strength and power to carry you through the day. Avoid white sugar, but go for honey.

7. Take Multivitamins Supplements

When your diets are lacking or because of destruction of vitamins and minerals during cooking, add multivitamins capsule or tablets to your meal, to supplement for missing vitamins and minerals.

Make sure that you consume magnesium daily, to enable you do physical work without having a higher rate of oxygen and heart beat. If you eat the above foods and nuts daily you would have enough of all minerals needed.

8.   Daily Consume Diets Made up of 90% – 95% of Fruits and Vegetables

It is recommended by experts that your daily meal should be made up of about 90 to 95 of fruits and vegetables. Eat dark green vegetables daily. Take oranges, apple, guava, paw-paw, pineapple, etc., daily.

9.   Avoid Harmful Habits Like Smoking, Caffeine, and Alcohol Intake.

The entire habits above are harmful to your health. It is even stated clearly in cigarette packs, that tobacco smoking is dangerous and that smokers may die young. You must quit smoking to look 20 years younger. Avoid caffeine and alcohol. As they contain harmful active components that are dangerous to health.

10.   Manage or Reduce Your Stress Level

Stress is usually brought about by fear, worry, anxiety, and anger. These things drain your energy, leaving you tired, haggard, and looking old. Learn to be quiet and relax well. Avoid tension or tense conditions.

11.   Drink at least Eight to Ten Glasses of Water Daily

Drinking up to eight glasses of water daily would help keep you hydrated and not dehydrated, which will cause you to look old and worn out.

You can start with two glasses of water in the morning immediately you wake up from bed, one glass before and after each three meals of a day.

If you do not eat three meals a day, you can still work it out. Water will also keep hunger pangs away from you.

12.   Take Snacks Between Meals if Necessary

You can snack on some fruit when you feel like eating between meals, to help feel your stomach and reduce hunger pangs. Instead of snacking on biscuits, cakes, and other pastries, snack on fruits and little of yogurt and nuts.

13. Do Medical Checkup

If you have anemia or any body weakness, consult a doctor and make sure that your blood is diagnosed to find out underlying causes of anemia or any other disease plaguing you, and to find cure or take all necessary medication to rejuvenate your body. This will enable you to be healthy and look younger.

Five Top Tips for Living a Stress Free Life

Stress symptoms include physical, social and mental indicators. Such symptoms include headache, sleeplessness and over-sleeping, extreme exhaustion and loss of appetite or over-appetite. Stress can be managed to the extent of living a stress free life, all through the year.

Stress is a state of high tension or pressure impacting hardship. In Simple understanding, stress is anything that disturbs the natural balance between the body and the environment.

Stress management is the ability to maintain control when people, situations, circumstances and events, try to make excessive demands on an individual, almost to a breaking point.

The following top tips for living a stress free life would help you manage, control and prevent stress with ease:

1. Have A Good Health Education.

A good health education would enable you to have an insight into your various stress triggers and then devise a means of freedom or a means of coping with it.

2. Always live on the positive side of Life.

For you to cope with or manage stress, to the extend of being stress free, you must always think positive, speak positive, act positive and live positive.

You must have nothing to do with worry and anxiety, in every form of situation.

3. Live A Healthy Live Daily.

To live a tress free life all through the year, you must think health and do the following:

i. Eat Balanced Diets.

Eat more of vegetables and fruits, up to 90% of your daily diet. They are full of minerals and vitamins, to help keep you energetic, strong and vibrant.

ii. Do Daily and Regular Exercise.

When you wake up from bed, stretch yourself, do jogging, go swimming, walk some distance, lift weights, do deep breathing daily, for about five minutes.

ii. Stop Or Avoid Harmful Habits.

Habits such as smoking of cigarette, drinking of alcohol and excess of caffeine are harmful to your health. Also, avoid self medication. These harmful habits often bring about stress. Get rid of them.

4. Be Free From Fear.

Do not be afraid what tomorrow may bring. Each morning, look up and move on through the day. In every situation, do not panic, just gain the control and you shall overcome.

5. Observe Good Attitudes Daily.

Your lifestyle must change in order to become stress free. As such, the following good attitudes should be observed:

i) Put A Demand On Relaxation Daily, ii) Learn to communicate well, iii) Make contacts and friends, iv) Do something for others, v) Learn to smile and laugh too, to enable you release yourself, these when done would help you get your mind off yourself and your situations.

6. Get Enough Sleep.

Lack of sleep can bring about or worsen stress. You must sleep for eight (8) hours daily. Sleeping these hours enables your body to be refreshed and stress daily.

The services of a doctor or a professional counselor can be made use of, when you realize that stress is too hard on you.

CHAPTER 5

Exercise, Fitness, and Health

Various exercise, fitness, and health measures are necessary to becoming a healthier and younger looking.

Eight Simple Ways to Flatten Your Tummy and Look Younger

Living a life with a bloated tummy portrays one as having no knowledge of what to do, in order to avoid, flatten, or control one's stomach.

Though many things may result in a bloated tummy, there are simple ways in which one can use to flatten his or her stomach, in order to remain or look younger.

These simple ways are as follows:

1. Drink 8 – 10 Glasses of Water Daily.

Drinking lots of water daily would help to flush your system of clogs and impurities. So, drink lots of water daily, up to 8 – 10 glasses.

Drinking much water daily, would make you to eat less food. This is so because; the water would reduce hunger pangs, which would have caused you to eat much.

Much water helps in digestion, thereby removing the problem of a bloated tummy. Lots of water taken daily would help to flush any bloating your experience.

2. Avoid or Stop the intake of Alcohol.

Alcohol is dangerous to your health. Medical report say that alcohol causes bloating of tummy, due to its ability to cause the accumulation of fat in the stomach, by raising cortisol levels in the body.

Alcohol is also known to dehydrate the body, leaving patches of bloats in tummy.

3. Consume More Fiber Daily.

Fiber in your diets would help prevent bloating due to constipation. Fiber diets also help to reduce your weight, including tummy weight gain.

Cut down your intake of carbohydrates, such as white bread and white rice. To get fiber you need, take vegetables, fruits, brown, and whole wheat bread.

4. Eat Balanced and Small Portions of Food or Meals.

Eat small portions of food or meals throughout the day, than eating 2 - 3 big portions. Smaller portions eaten many times a day would help digestion to take place faster, to avoid giving your tummy a bloated look.

Eat healthy snacks like almonds every morning and night, which help in burning fat, and sometimes just take desserts, all these helps to flatten your tummy.

Consume calcium diets or take it as a daily supplement of 1000mg to 1200mg.

This would help keep your bones strong, and avoid fractured bones that cause slump looks. Avoid much intake of whole milk, it causes bloating of the tummy.

5. Engage in Daily Regular Exercise.

Exercise for 30 minutes to one hour indoors and 30 minutes to one hour outdoor daily or five times a week. Go jogging, swimming, brisk walking, and running. Do weight lifting, bench press to build your chest, and practice perfect posture exercises.

Also, always sit and stand straight. Never slump when sitting down. Be active daily. Exercise would help your system to be able to burn fat faster, thereby eliminating the problem of a bloated tummy.

6. Do Deep Breathing Daily.

Make sure that you do deep breathing for about 5 minutes daily. This should involve breathing from your abdomen, and not from your chest.

So, try to take the deep breath from your lower abdomen. This would help to pull your tummy back and help the burning of fat.

7. Avoid a stressful Life.

Medical report say that too much of stress results in increases in levels of a hormone, called cortisol levels, thus enabling fat to be sent to the stomach.

You must manage stress appropriately. Learn to rest well and eliminate stressful activities.

8. Quit or Stop Smoking.

As in stress, smoking is also reported to raise levels of cortisol. This causes smokers to have increases in abdominal fat, thus a bloated tummy.

As you seek to flatten your tummy, do not give up easily, just follow the above tips, and you shall get a flattened tummy that gives you fitness and a younger look you desire.

Exercise and Healthy Living

Being healthy involves a number of things of which exercise has to be considered. The following tips would help you become healthy, as you put them into practice:

Exercise aims at maintaining at giving fitness, health, strong bones, weight loss and a general well-being. When exercise is done properly, in addition to rest, sleep, and good diet, it brings desired goals.

Exercise comes in different forms, such as jogging, swimming, bicycle riding, weight lifting, walking, jump rope type, etc. All categories of persons are expected to perform one exercise or the other based on their state of health.

Some persons who are diabetic need to seek the approval of a medical doctor for help in exercising, to avoid injury.

Exercise has been proved through research to give great benefits to the body, such as

i) Putting up strong bones

ii) Gives a healthy weight, by removing excess fat in the body

iii) Reduction in the risk of some illnesses like diabetes, hypertension, and cancer

iv) Exercise is shown to improve one's self-worth and much more.

v)

When one is able to go on with the activities of the day without stress, such can say fitness is into play. At this time the body is strong and able to carry out various activities, and being immune to most infections, like common cold.

Physical fitness comes to stay when such factors like muscle strength, flexibility, muscle endurance, body composition, and cardio-respiratory endurance comes into play.

Exercise is so important that all need to have it on a daily basis, to be able to significantly improve their quality of life.

As a rule, it is recommended that one has to get exercise for 15 – 30 minutes at a time, without stopping, to be able to profit optimally.

You must exercise sufficiently to increase your pulse rate to about two third your maximum heart rate. This level must also be maintained for 15-30 minutes without stopping.

However, when stopping, one should observe a cooling down period. That is doing and not just to stop abruptly, it can be dangerous, when the heart is beating heavily. When about to stop abruptly, slow down your speed or heart beat rate, by slowing down the activity or exercise.

Research has shown that even brisk walking alone can still be beneficial, and may add to one's life span.

Exercising outdoors by brisk walking to stretch out one's legs, at least once a week, is seen to be beneficial, when discipline is taken seriously.

Exercise and Good Nutrition for Healthier Living

Good diet or nutrition and exercise are going to go along together for our bodies. Exercise is going to give us fitness along with four major things:

flexibility, strength, muscle endurance, and cardiovascular health. Diet on its own is not going to be able to give you this.

You need to have the physical part as well. One thing to remember is that a bad diet can affect the way that your fitness training goes even if you follow the best type of exercise plan that you can.

You need to put a healthy diet and a lot of exercise together to stay as healthy as you can.

How long do you need to exercise to keep as healthy as you can? The average is at least 20 minutes of exercise at least three times a week.

This will help to strengthen the cardiovascular health. Another idea is that 3500 calories must be used in a week by doing any sort of physical activity.

This will benefit you and your heart as well. It is a good idea to speak to your doctor first to find out what exercise plan is going to be best for you and your body.

The energy nutrients that are stored like glucose and fatty acids with a few amino acids are let out into the blood during exercise in order to provide energy for what you are doing.

This means that the body will respond to exercise by adjusting its fuel amounts.

Experts have made a way to use diet to control high blood pressure and now they are finding out that exercise has a role in keeping blood pressure from increasing.

With the reduction of sodium into your body, weight loss and limited alcohol use, along with the increased amount of physical activity and a low fat diet, you can control hypertension.

Foods that are used for the purpose of lowering blood pressure without using medication can include sweets and many beverages that have sugar in them, red meat and fats.

To build muscle in the body, proteins are used and this is true when the body is at rest after exercise or any type of physical activity.

There is research that has shown that athletes will retain more protein and use more of it as fuel for the body. The American Dietetic Association has said that one gram per kilogram of body weight is recommended for people that do not exercise at all.

For the athletes, the protein amounts are going to be higher. It should be considered that athletes also need more carbohydrates as well. If they do not take in enough carbohydrates, their protein will be used all up for fuel and there will not be anything left for muscle building after exercise is done.

Researches say that weight bearing exercises like walking, dancing, running, sports and so much more, are very good at getting good bone health.

Eating disorders like bulimia and anorexia have been said to damage bone strength. Exercise alone cannot make your body healthy.

You need to have the proper calcium and other vitamins and minerals required for bones must go with the adequate amount of exercise to provide the best bone health.

Along with exercise, diet can help keep your body working good and in the right mode for the rest of your life.

How to Perform Natural Deep Breathing Exercise

This write up provides information about breathing, shows how natural deep breathing improves health, and gives ways of properly engaging in natural deep breathing.

To benefit from natural deep breathing, follow the steps below:

1. Know The Benefits Of Deep Breathing.

If you have not read my article on health benefits of deep breathing, you can check it out after, but here is a brief list that have been established by doctors and experts in natural deep breathing:

a. Through deep breathing the diaphragm moves downward and massages the stomach, liver, and other organs below it. Also, when it moves upwards, it massages the heart.

b. The upward and downward movement of the diaphragm detoxifies your inner organs and promotes blood flow.

c. Deep Breathing helps to pump the lymph more efficiently through the lymphatic system, which is part of our immune system.

ci.

d. Natural deep breathing helps in reducing stress in our lives.

di.

e. Natural deep breathing improves our general health.

f. Deep breathing increases vitality, promotes relaxation and prolongs longevity

2. How to Perform Natural Deep Breathing

The technique of natural deep breathing is easy to understand. When you must have understood the technique, you can then begin to benefit from natural deep breathing.

To understand and do the exercise, follow the tips below:

i. Start your fitness exercise with natural deep breathing

ii. Seek a quiet and comfortable place that is void of distraction.

iii. Lie down, sit down, or stand.

Just take a posture that is comfortable to you.

iv. Avoid tension and negative emotions

Get your mind and muscles in a state of relaxation, to avoid having shallow breathing.

v. Inhale slowly and deeply, right from your lower abdomen, through your nostrils.

vi. Hold the breath while counting silently and slowly to 10 or just a count of 10 seconds.

vii. Exhale deeply with your mouth and nostrils open.

Make sure that you empty your lungs completely during this time.

viii. As you exhale, count to 5 or to a period of 5 seconds.

ix. Do or repeat the exercise for about 5 minutes or more, as stated above.

Remember to avoid distractions during this time, by concentrating your mind and physical being to the exercise only.

x. You must carryout this practice on a daily basis and regularly.

xi.

The above process is what you need to start enjoying and reaping the manifold health benefits of natural deep breathing.

Nine Health Benefits of Natural Deep Breathing Exercise

Many experts in deep breathing exercise agree that there are numerous benefits that follow those who engage in deep breathing exercise.

Deep breathing has immense benefits to your health and has much effect in promoting longevity or life span.

Once the routine of deep breathing is started and continued, you would begin to reap immense benefits from its exercise.

The following stated benefits which experts in deep breathing have researched and acclaimed, would help you understand its importance and need for you to engage in the exercise:

1. Relaxation of Bowels

Deep breathing helps to relax your bowels. When trying to move your bowels in the toilet, deep breathing would enable you do so easily. While sitting on the toilet bowl, do deep breathing and your bowels would move.

2. Stress Reliever

Deep breathing relieves stress. Stress is injurious to health. Usually, the gross activities of a day, coupled with other factors, can bring about stress. But deep breathing works on your system, making it possible for you to be free from stress or less prone to stress.

3. Improves and Increases Oxygen Delivery and Supply to Body Organs

Deep breathing from the tummy helps provide an optimal supply of oxygen to all your body organs.

When deep breathing is routinely done, it both improves and increases delivery and level of oxygen supplied to body organs. This enables your system to do better.

4. Improves the Detoxification of body Organs and Cleanses the Body

Deep breathing, when done regularly, helps in the improvement of detoxification of body organs.

When harmful poisons or toxins accumulate in the body, they cause harm. But deep breathing helps in the elimination of these toxins, and thus cleanses the body.

5. Deep Breathing Releases you from Anxiety

Deep breathing would help clear every clog in your mind, giving you a focused life, and thus releasing and relieving you from anxiety. Anxiety is dangerous to your health, and can cause many health problems and diseases.

6. Deep Breathing Promotes your Well-being

Deep breathing helps your system to release certain hormones that help to give you a sense of good health and well-being, relaxing your muscles. Thus, you get relief from muscle tension and pain.

7. Deep breathing improves your Physical and Mental Health

Your physical well-being is bound to improve as you engage in regular deep breathing. Also, your mental alertness improves, making it possible for you to be able to do what you could not do before.

8. Deep Breathing Helps to Lower your Blood Pressure

High blood pressure is that which many dread. With routine and regular deep breathing exercises, your blood pressure becomes lowered. Thus, bring your blood pressure to an approved level.

9. Deep Breathing Can Relief you from Nervousness

Nervousness and the inability to speak due to fear or nervousness can be relieved with the use of deep breathing.

The key to success in deep breathing is regular and routine exercise. When you learn the ropes of deep breathing, apply them, and you shall reap all the above benefits.

Boost Your Health with Regular Exercise

Expert researches and studies, say that regular exercise is very important, and has health benefits.

The following health benefits of exercise would help you get the best out of regular exercise.

1. Regular exercise improves the quality and duration of sleep.

Your sleep becomes sweet with regular exercise. The inability to sleep would be taken away. When you wake up, you would not experience fatigue. You would have a better night rest, wake up strong, and active.

2. Regular exercise reduces anxiety and depression.

Vigorous exercise done regularly reduces feelings of anger, depression, and confusion.

It takes you to a high point, whereby anxiety diminishes, depression vanishes, and you put on a feeling of good health. Exercise is known to improve your mood, leaving no room for depression moods.

To be free from anxiety, get regular exercise, such as bicycle riding, jogging, and brisk walking around.

Researches found that exercising for 20 to one hour, three times a week, diminishes depression.

3. Regular exercise refreshes, invigorates, and improves health.

Your blood flow would improve. Oxygen and nutrients supply to your brain improves, thereby giving you mental alertness, and ability to think better.

4. Regular exercise relieves stress.

Jogging, swimming, and brisk walking can help relief stress and give you a positive outlook and life. You become physically fit, emotionally sound, and mentally alert.

Stress breaks down your body's immune system and makes you vulnerable to common infections like common colds, etc, and memory impairment.

5. Regular exercise helps boost your sense of self-worth.

Engaging in exercises that stretch and strengthen you, makes you feel better and able to face the world. Exercising regular would help to uplift your self-worth, imparting in you the 'I can do' courage.

6. Regular exercise gives your mind needed time out from daily responsibility and duties.

7. Regular exercise strengthens your bones, and opens your chest.

Your joints, legs, hands, bones, spines, and chest, become strengthened as you engage in exercise.

Your posture would improve. Your chest would open, allowing you to have deep regular breathing that your body needs.

8. Regular exercise takes pains away.

Pains that often come with waking up in the morning, and the weakness that follow, would go with regular exercise.

9. Regular exercise would help you cut down on excess weight, and give you that fitness and health you need.

10. Regular exercise imparts and impacts vigor, youthfulness, and beauty in your look and life.

With the above benefits of regular exercise, in mind, there is need to discipline yourself and engage in regular exercise on a daily basis, to be able to reap the benefits that follow.

Best Exercise for Fitness and Health

Exercise is very important for the human body. Lots of exercise is known to dissolve many disorders of the body. This happens when on engages in vigorous exercise.

As you continue in the degree of your exercise, infections like common colds subside, diseases that are degenerative in nature disappear, life quality improves, and life span increases.

To understand which exercise is best for fitness and health, consider the following points:

1. Competitive sports are not the best form of exercise for certain ages.

Competitive sports should remain with the youths. But when it comes to time when the body really needs exercise, when one has attained the age of 35 and above, this is when exercise is beneficial and required.

At this time, you should start exercising for better life. This is because; your health would begin to deteriorate during this time, if you refuse to give attention to exercise.

This deterioration in health usually occurs because you are no more interested in competitive sports, and aging.

2. Characteristics of Best Exercise.

Best exercise should be characterized by vigorous workouts and should be non-violent. For example, running and jogging.

You must maintain a high level of athletic training, to make running and jogging safe. If you have no training, limit yourself to non-violent exercises like walking, and then get training for vigorous exercises, for your improve quality of life.

3. Non-Competitive Sports or Best Exercise.

You must get training or learn the sport that is non-competitive. This is sport that can be enjoyed alone. Start out with 30 minutes daily, and move on to about one hour daily.

Spend this time in vigorous exercise outdoor. Also, spend another 30 minutes to about one hour daily indoor, in such activities that require muscular energy to be expended.

Your physical condition and fitness would be better when you get involved in these vigorous exercises.

4. Why you must Exercise Vigorously.

a. This type of exercise is the secret behind your having vigor, youthfulness, and beauty. Just take your exercise seriously. Start jogging in the morning and in the evening, if you are chanced, and reap the benefits.

b. This type of exercise would keep you in good shape and active too. Make exercise, part of your daily routine activity.

c. If you are a beginner in exercise, you may get the services of a trainer or professional to supervise what you do. That means you pay to get the best result.

d. You would become alert, fit, and healthy as you exercise. Exercise would help you cut down and maintain your weight. If you fail to exercise, you would start putting on weight.

e. Get involved also with swimming.

When you swim, you exercise some major muscles of your body. Some persons classify swimming as their number one exercise.

To stay fit, healthy, and happy, daily give yourself a dose of vigorous exercise that you enjoy doing.

Five Ways to Lose Weight

Here are the top most and easy methods of reducing weight, without stress or unnecessary expenditure.

Getting on with life and having a balanced diet on a daily basis is the desire for many. Living without this, is the result of most people being over-weight.

Below are tested methods or tips in which appreciable results have been obtain in shedding away unwanted weight gain.

1. Do not skip breakfast.

Make sure that you get up early enough each day, so as not to miss your daily breakfast. This is very important because breakfast is both good for your health and getting rid of excess weight.

Breakfast would help your body to accept food throughout the day. Make sure that you keep boiled eggs in your fridge and some high fiber, low starch fruits too in your fridge.

You may decide to eat fruits all through the day, but do not forget to start that with breakfast.

2. Drink About 8 – 10 Glasses of Water Daily.

You can become used to this by starting out first thing in the morning. You can take 2 glasses immediately after waking from sleep, first thing in the morning before eating food.

This can help create an aware of the need to make up the remaining glasses through the day. Water is not bitter, so you must try and drink it first in the morning.

3. Do Physical Exercise Daily and Regularly

Exercise can help you reduce weight and also maintain it. When you wake up stretch your hands, legs, neck, and body. Breathe in and out for about five minutes at a time.

You can also do some work up like weight lifting, jogging, jumping, etc This should be done daily and regularly in the morning.

4. Avoid Junk Food.

Make sure that you avoid these foods that are called fast foods and such others like sweets, cakes, fried foods, and snacks. Eat much of fruits.

Your diet such contain more of fruits tan carbohydrates. Get oranges, melons, grapes, etc.

5. Eat Enough Of Vegetables Daily.

You need vegetables to get enough fiber in your diet. If you have stop eating vegetables daily, start doing so regularly.

You can look out in cookery books for their recipes and enjoy yourself.

Your weight loss is very important for having a healthy body and living a long life, so get involved in the necessary methods and shed that extra weight.

Knowing and doing the above would certainly lead to one becoming happier, healthier and younger looking.

To your healthier and younger looking life.

www.ingramcontent.com/pod-product-compliance
Lightning Source LLC
Chambersburg PA
CBHW070653290526
45790CB00001B/304